Stand, Step, & Walk Yourself to a Healthier You

I0440120

Daniel Paul D'Aniello

About this E-Book

I love fitness and overall health. My search has involved seeking for the balance of physical fitness and nutrition. From weight lifting, to running, to yoga, to home exercise DVDs, I have tried it all in the pursuit of my own physical wellbeing.

Studies have shown that while regular and more intense exercise is important for overall health, the simple act of standing and walking can have amazing, long lasting, and permanent positive impacts on managing weight, health, and overall happiness.

What if the simple act of putting one foot in front of the other can slow down aging, help maintain a healthy weight, boost positive mood, ignite brain activity, and train the cardiovascular system to perform at its best?

This ebook seeks to promote healthier living by advocating that standing up and walking can have numerous positive health benefits. It further provides personal experience and practical advise for the sedentary or moderately active individual of all ages.

In the end, we are the best stewards of our own health.

Join me in a journey of self-improvement and simplicity.

Put one foot in front of the other and stand, step, and walk yourself to a healthier you.

Dedication

This ebook is dedicated to the many wonderful health professionals who have helped increase our understanding of human health and fitness.

This ebook is also dedicated to all people who feel that life can feel uncontrollable at times.

Here's to seizing control of our lives by taking simple steps to improve our health, mental outlook and always pursuing our very best life.

Disclaimer

This ebook has been written and designed to provide helpful information for individuals looking to live a healthier lifestyle. The information presented and opinions shared, are based on the author's experience and knowledge obtained from his own reading, research, and experience.

The author is not a medical professional, nutritionist, or a fitness instructor. He intends to provide valuable information for the overall purpose of inspiring, motivating, and driving people to find their own reasons to improve their health.

Readers of this e-book are encouraged to conduct their own research, understand their own bodies, and consult with their own medical providers before embarking on any strenuous or dramatic lifestyle changes or pursuing any of the recommendations made in this ebook.

Other eBooks by Daniel Paul D'Aniello
Available on Amazon.com

The iStudent and iTeacher: A Revolution Unfolding

Learning and Loving Doggie Style – How Dogs Can Be Our Life Gurus

Flames of Religious Passion in Brooklyn: Scandal and Religious Liberty in 19th C Oneida Community Brooklyn

Hit a Home Run in AP US History on Day One

End the Elephant – The Argument to End the Republican Party and Replace it with a National Liberty Party

Contents

1. Introduction
My journey to standing up, stepping, and walking myself healthier

I have fond and vibrant memories of my youth. Born to two terrific and caring parents hailing from a little town near Sorrento, Italy, I had a typical childhood of a first generation American. My sister and I were raised with love and laughter. But I never gave much thought to my health, as most young people do. I thought myself to be young, free, and free of the restrictions of monitoring my health and fitness. As a child, I was within the normal weight range for my age. And then it happened. As I entered middle school, I began to amass unwanted pounds on my frame.

The gain was gradual and crept up on me. Before I knew it, I was wearing size 44-waist and was well over 200 pounds! Just the thought of my past self sends shivers down my spine... Despite my heavy state, I was not as aware of my size as I should have been.

Coming from an Italian family, food was always plentiful and tantalized the taste buds. How could I say no to a delicious bowl of freshly made pasta with from scratch tomato sauce (no self respecting Italian uses the stuff found in markets) sprinkled with heavenly bits of parmigiano cheese – accompanied with a half a loaf of sesame studded bread to wipe up all that scrumptiousness? I had no care of calories from fat, carbs, portion sizes, or the temporary blissful but calorically dangerous excursions into the world of dessert. Along with my savory tooth, I was also blessed (and cursed) with a sweet one. I could never finish a meal without something sweet, gooey, decadent, or creamy. Consequently, this is one desire that I still fight with the most. As I gained weight, I became less physically active and continued my eating without cause for concern.

There were many moments during that time that cause me to shiver still to this day. Like the one time that my Mom, in a valiant attempt to increase my physical activity and socialization, brought my sister and I to gymnastics class. The instructor was thrilled at the prospect of two new pupils but lacked modern day tact when it comes to protecting the self-esteem of a young boy. This wonderful man (not in particularly good shape himself) took one look at me, jiggled my protruding abdomen and proclaimed, "Well, at least being here will help you lose some of that mozzarella!"

I was mortified. Suffice it to say that I refused to make a second visit to that fool of a man. This painful memory is one that has long remained with me. On a personal note, I find that the damage adults do to the minds of young people can sometimes be inadvertent, but long lasting to say the least. My father always told me, "If you have nothing nice to say, then say nothing." It's advice that I struggle to follow with adults (although we should have a little thicker skin), but I am very cautious of potential damaging remarks to young children or people. When I was a high school teacher, I tried very hard to be aware of my students' feelings. A friend of mine was dealt a painful memory when her grandmother used to tease her about her weight as a child. Anyone caring for or interacting with children should watch their tongue. That gymnastics man who hurled his mozzarella insult at me hurt my confidence although I overcame that, the memory still lingers...

But I digress – back to my tale.

My low point in my eating habits came during a typical event in a private school child's experience: a chocolate fundraiser. I had to get rid of a box of chocolate bars. I brought the box into my room. Day after day, the prospect of going out in the neighborhood, ringing doorbells to sell chocolate bars didn't appeal to me (Never mind the fact that my neighborhood was at least half comprised of Orthodox Jews, of whom would not buy my chocolate). Sloth and gluttony collided and propelled a fateful decision – one that was my rock bottom point in my relationship with health, fitness, and food...

So, in an act of gluttony (and brilliance I must admit) I decided that I would gradually get rid of that chocolate by selling it to a great customer: myself. Each day after school I would go home and after having had a snack in the kitchen, I would go upstairs into my room. After all, there was a job to be done! The chocolate had to be sold. So I would grab a dollar, place it in the box, take a bar (sometimes two) and enjoy the wonderful and addictive experience of consuming velvety smooth chocolate. Everyone was happy: the school got its pound of flesh, I completed my task, and every day I got to enjoy some chocolate.

Horrible isn't it? At the time, I didn't think anything wrong with it but today; I am stunned at my action. For the longest time, I kept this dirty secret. Few people actually know of this shameful event from my past. But now, I wear it as my very own scarlet letter: "G" for gluttony. I should probably add "S" for sloth as well. This sad tale is my own experience using food as a comfort and shield against the world. How many of us use food as a psychological crutch? Oh how those French fries can numb the pain of loneliness. How many of us use the soothing creaminess of ice cream to temper our anger? There must be many Americans who have been guilty at one time or another using food as an emotional Novocain – a powerful numbing agent for our daily troubles.[1]

But then, a confluence of events led to a transformation. As I ended my sophomore year of high school I had a realization: I wasn't happy being fat. I think that the typical high school pressures of looking good and being attractive eventually shook up my complacency. So, I undertook a relatively easy routine: each day I would skip lunch. While not the smartest or most healthy way to lose weight, the decreased caloric intake did the trick (and this simple insight is perhaps one of the most powerful one). I must admit that it took a great deal of willpower to do this. Even when I got home each day with a pounding headache from that empty stomach, I wouldn't snack. I wouldn't eat until dinner and even then I ate my usual portion – nothing more.

Well, junior year was my best physically speaking and in terms of my grades. I looked and felt better than I ever had. My confidence soared. Still, I knew that the weight loss could be reversed and so I sought out ways to get into better shape and stay that way. I asked my parents for one of those home weight-lifting machines and they graciously agreed. And while I never really achieved 8% body fat (that's still one of my top fitness goals), the regular workouts kept the weight at bay. For the rest of my teenage years and into my twenties, I would perform weight lifting and cardio work on a treadmill.

My thirties brought another surprise. Once again, my weight had ballooned. I continued to exercise daily for about 30 minutes but that no longer seemed to work. My food portions grew once more into gargantuan proportions. My metabolism was slowing as I got a little older. I needed something else.

Today, I have found my secret to keeping my weight into a normal range for my height. I follow a daily routine of food tracking through Weight Watchers, high intensity exercise, frequent standing, and by stepping/walking an average of 17,000-20,000 steps a day. And this change demanded that I make a personal vow: no more weight loss yo-yos. I will live a lifestyle that will keep me in the best shape possible!

Why did I tell you of my life's food and health trials? Because I want you to know that like many Americans, I have and continued to battle the constant need to eat more than I should and not move around as much as I should.

But standing, stepping, and walking is the focus of this ebook. We all know the value of portion control, getting our fruits/veggies, and exercising. But are we as focused on practicing an active lifestyle in which we stand around and just walk? Are Americans aware how powerful standing up and walking around really are to health? Are doctors, government officials, and health insurance companies doing enough to motivate people to not only eat well, exercise, but to get up and move? Have we gotten so wrapped up in our work, families, and entertainment that we have forgotten the basic tool we all have available to get healthy?

I believe so.

But I also believe that by understanding the basics and reconnecting with the simple act of walking all people can reclaim their right and responsibility to a healthy life.

The character Blanche Devereaux in the hit 90s comedy *The Golden Girls*, once remarked to her roommates: "I treat my body like a temple." I think we all should adopt that philosophy when it comes to our health.

Let's treat our bodies like temples. Lets build them, nurture them, and maintain them. With a healthy eating plan, moderate physical exercise, and simple walking we all can improve our temples.

Let us begin.

Stand, step, and walk yourself to a healthier you.

2. America the Unhealthy
A snapshot of Americans' health problems

Before we can take our journey, we should understand the root of our problems. Americans simply are not active enough. We eat way too much and move way too little. And much of this is born of our desire for greater comfort and business interests that want to make it easier and faster for consumers to consume. Heavy reliance on cars, technology, drive-thrus, processed food, fast food, convenience, and increased demands on one's time help create this massive problem. I am keenly aware that for some people, this diagnosis is too simplistic. But for the majority who face no physical disability or genetic predisposition to gaining weight, we have to look ourselves in the mirror. And we have to understand that our choices are having horrible impacts on our health, our families, our communities, and our society at large.

How many Americans are obese? According to the Center for Disease Control (CDC), 35.7% of Americans are obese.[2] A third of the nation is obese! Roughly 100 million Americans are in this category of having too much weight for their height. Obesity is measured by weight or more commonly by one's body mass index (BMI). Using BMI, health officials can use objective data (a person's height and weight) to determine whether or not that person is technically below normal weight, at normal weight, overweight, obese, or morbidly obese. And while BMI may not be the most exact measurement to determine whether one is overweight or not (due to variables such as body composition), it is the most commonly used method of determining ideal body weight for most people. Here's an easy web-based BMI calculator.

I am still struck by the fact that a third of Americans are obese. These are not Americans who have just a few pounds to lose. How and why have we reached this point? Sedentary lifestyles, too much technology, and poor eating habits are primarily to blame. Obesity causes so much pain for the individual, for families, and for communities. It places stress on the healthcare system as obesity has a cascading effect on so many other aspects of health. In 2008, the estimated economic cost of obesity in the United States was $147 billion dollars![3] That economic drain has places a tremendous burden on doctors, patients, and the healthcare system.

How do we begin to address such a problem that continues to plague our modern lives? Because if we do not, then more and more Americans will suffer an increasing array of physical and emotional ailments as a result. A huge part of the answer lies within making lifestyle choices that are harmonious with a healthy body.

Heart disease is another weight on America's health problems. Again, the CDC states that 600,000 Americans die each hear due to heart disease.[4] And once again, a contributing culprit to this terrible scientific fact is that being overweight is caused by overeating and a sedentary lifestyle. So many lives are touched by heart disease and millions of dollars are spent in an attempt to deal with the problem once it has reared its ugly head. Still, prevention is key to tackling this tremendous problem and so many of the chronic illnesses and disorders affecting millions of Americans.

Obesity and heart disease are just the tip of the iceberg when it comes to America's health problems. Scientific studies are showing how dozens and dozens of health ailments are caused by lack of physical activity, such as high blood pressure, increased levels of anxiety and emotional issues, and certain cancers.[5] Despite these very real dangers, there are simple ways to combat them. And other studies show that movement and exercise can activate the body's own defense mechanisms against cancer.[6] It is high time that we do more to combat this problem of epidemic proportions.

Fortunately, the answer lies in a rather simple formula: move more and eat less. I'll explore both elements to this elixir of a healthy life in the chapters to follow. With greater education and by adapting healthier lifestyles, we can begin to turn the tide against many of these costly ailments.

3. Why Step?
The current thinking on why standing and stepping can overhaul your health

Fitness trends and workouts come and go, but walking is simple, portable, and constant way to improve health. The mere act of standing up and walking provides a myriad of scientifically measured benefits. By standing up you increase the electrical activity in your body. You can activate your metabolism. Your body regulates hormones more effectively – unleashing a cascade of positive affects on your body and mind. You can feel better, you can think more clearly, and you can live a better and healthier life.

There are many obstacles for us to get up and walk. The human body was made to move. For millennia, people would walk numerous miles a day in addition to performing physical activity. Surviving required the ability to build and maintain a dwelling and obtaining food either by hunting or farming (personally, I don't miss the days of having to farm or hunt for my food but do miss the natural physical demands that would require).

Today, technology and our lifestyles have contributed to the decline of walking and standing. Many people spend their entire workdays in a chair sitting at a desk. There are studies that show this lack of activity is perhaps a great contributor to physical maladies then we had previously thought.[7] Couple that with tremendous advances and availability of food supply and increasingly large portions of what people eat, it's not a surprise why people across the globe are getting heavier and unhealthier.

The "sitting disease" is making things even worse for maintaining a healthy lifestyle. Go watch a movie for two hours and you'll be shutting down your body's activity. Watch television and chances are you will be sitting for half hour an hour or maybe even more. And if you work in the office as many people do, chances are you are sitting at a desk for a large percentage of your working time. Tom Rath, author of *Eat Move Sleep*, Has written extensively about this modern-day problem. In fact, he suggests that sitting is one the primary causes of unhealthy living by most Americans today. Rath writes, "Sitting is the most underrate health threat of modern times. This subtle epidemic is eroding our health. On a global level, inactivity now kills more people than smoking."[8] Truly, this was an alarm for me.

As I read his book, I became more anxious than ever about my own daily habits. Rath sounds the alarm that sitting shuts down the electrical muscles in your legs which then sets off a chain reaction in the body: calories burned drops to one per minute, fat busting enzyme production drops 90 percent, and even levels of good cholesterol decrease after two hours of sitting. Sitting down powers down the body.

This information provoked my thinking and helped challenge my beliefs. When I was younger, I believed that my daily half hour or even hour workouts were sufficient to keep me healthy and control my weight. But despite exercising daily, I still maintained more weight than I should have. One key to increasing your level of fitness is to avoid inactivity as much as possible.

Isn't it a wonder despite the increase in knowledge of fitness, health, and nutrition, Americans are still getting fatter and unhealthier? I was walking around in a department store and from the corner of my eye, I saw very large woman strolling along. Now, I'm trying not to look down upon people who are heavier. After all, I was one of these people at one time. But I could not help asking myself why this person was so heavy? Was she lazy? Did she eat too much? Did she exercise at all? Is she genetically predisposed those two holding onto weight? I couldn't answer any of these questions. But it was obvious that this woman was the beyond the normal range for her height. The ironic part of it all is that the reason why I went this department store was because the weather outside is raining and I want to walk around. This simple trick of strolling around and department stores is a very easy way to increase your physical activity without sacrificing much at all. I'll elaborate on this little trick and others later.

Getting back to the heavy lady in the department store, I cannot help but believe that this woman would do her herself an immense amount of good by walking around more frequently (ironically, she was). Grant it, I have no awareness of her own unique personal obstacles in managing her weight. I'll try to stay away from the judgmental aspect of her outward appearance. But I am a firm believer that this woman (and so many people) can find healthier living by standing, stepping, and walking. Being healthy is not just about looking good and adhering to social norms of fitness. It's about creating the best quality of life for you. And through my experience, I am convinced that anything you can do to enhance your physical health is a blessing. In United States, healthcare costs are soaring. Billions of dollars could be saved if more Americans seized control and took responsibility for their health. Rather than focus on health care insurance reforms and hospital reforms (while important) we should be focusing on the little things that can increase self-awareness and fitness and nutrition for all.

I love to exercise. I love using dumbbells, DVD workouts, running on the treadmill, and all different types of exercises. But I have found that one of the most effective simple and profound ways to positively impact your life and health is simple: stand up, step, and walk. I was doing some research and began reading about studies that show the importance of frequent and consistent physical movement. These studies support new focus on increasing daily movement. At some places of work, the rise of treadmill desks and standing desks at a place of employment is more proof of the importance of the simple act of standing and walking.[9] Fitness trackers can help create more awareness for individuals to get more active. There are so many ways to support a healthier and more active lifestyle.

What Standing/stepping/walking won't do

Now, walking and standing is a tremendously good habit to cultivate. Another powerful reason to begin this habit is that it can be the gateway to even better habits, food choices, and a healthier lifestyle. For someone who is relatively inactive, starting this habit would produce fast and dramatic results. However, walking, standing, and/or exercising alone will not transform you into a healthy individual. You must come to grips with fundamental truths: you must be aware of what you eat and how much you eat of it.

I have exercised ever since I've been 15 years old. But I was not aware of the types and amount of food that I was eating. The problem was the out of proportion amount of eating for my size. When I had begun using Weight Watchers® online tracker to get a handle on my portions, my father joked with me to just cut in half what I was already eating. Why pay a company to do what was so simple? Yes, he spoke the truth (which is something that I'll be forced to admit). We can learn so much from our parents and elders! I have come to believe that merely cutting out a quarter of what you eat a day can begin to make tremendous impact on your weight loss and overall health. Eventually as your food and fitness goals evolve you can become more precise. That is why I have used online tools such as Weight Watchers to assist me. There are some terrific and free apps/tools that can really jump start you on this quest to get a control over what the amounts are eating. That is the goal: to be aware of your portions and to reduce them. For example, prior to my food portion modification, my afternoon snack would be a bagel with peanut butter and jelly. Now at the time, I had no clue as to how many calories I was consuming, nor did I want to know. When I calculated the point value of that snack according to Weight Watchers®, I was shocked. That snack (so deliciously creamy, crunchy, and carb laden) took up nearly a third of the daily points that I was allowed to consume in order to begin to lose weight. My point is that no amount of exercise, walking, or standing will create the necessary calorie deficit that you need in order to lose weight. This is a simple, albeit difficult, truth to accept.

While I would recommend incorporating the daily stepping/walking/standing routine into your life immediately, you need to identify what your goals are in order to begin a weight loss and fitness program. There are so many factors to consider ranging from your current fitness level, potential health issues that may have to be overcome, weight loss goals, or fitness training.

So whatever your fitness and weight loss goals are, you can get a jumpstart on them by initiating a standing, walking, standing stepping routine. You must get your calories under control. If you are beginning from a starting point of relatively low physical activity, and this new habit will put you on the path to a healthier you.

4. How to Step
An easy guide to begin standing up and stepping your way to better health

---

Now for the easy but paradoxically hard part: actually beginning a standing stepping walking routine that you can stick with. I will get you started by sharing my habits that I have cultivated over years of living a healthier lifestyle. Some of these you might find easy, some difficult, and some might even seem obsessive (as some of my family and friends have told me). Nonetheless, I think you will agree that it's important to get started somewhere and at times we can learn how to make ourselves better by looking to what others have already done for themselves. I truly hope that these tips will motivate, encourage, inspire, sustain, and propel you to a healthier version of yourself.

1. Create the right mindset

Before increasing your standing, stabbing, and walking, you must decide on why you are doing what you are about to do. Any successful self-improvement begins with a solid mental preparation and understanding of the task at hand. My healthy lifestyle is driven by three goals: to look good, to feel good, and delay disease and age. I sacrifice food choices and choose to move daily in order to support these goals. You must do the same. You must delve into yourself and find the reason why you want to embark on this journey. I have found that the reasons are best to be your own. Find the reason(s) why you want to become healthier. Summon the willpower necessary to begin and sustain your effort. Find comfort in the discipline needed to solidify your habits. Once you have the proper mental preparation for this new task, you will find it much easier to stand, step, and walk yourself to healthier you.

2. Get a fitness tracker/pedometer

When I was a teacher, one of our professional development sessions was focused on measuring things or quantifying. The main idea: what gets measured, gets done. This simple thought can be a starting point for your life transformation, across all areas. But in your fitness life, measuring things keeps you motivated encourages you and can drive you forward toward your healthy goals. Depending on your comfort with technology, you can purchase a simple or a very advanced fitness tracker. Personally, I have had great success with digital fitness trackers. My favorite of all time is one made by FitBit.

Digital fitness trackers are devices that gather your physical activity and then upload them to a website which can then translate that data. This provides unique insight into your daily physical activity. These handy devils are wonderful and quite addictive. FitBit also allows you to connect with family, friends, and other healthy minded people. You can use each other as motivation to walk more, take up jogging, or even starting a running program. I even use it as a source of competition by seeing who can get in the most steps.

But the best part of these devices is that it will give you an immediate understanding of your physical activity or lack thereof. Note that there is a difference between intense exercising and adding standing, stepping, and walking to your daily routine. More on that to follow but for now, remember that what gets measured gets done!

3. Aim for 10,000 steps a day

Most studies suggest that Americans should aim for 10,000 steps a day.[10] That may seem a lot but it really isn't. It roughly translates to walking or running for a total of 5miles. But there are so many ways you can reach your 10,000. Once you get your fitness tracker, I recommend observing your normal daily routine and see where you are. Many fitness experts cite anything under 6,000 steps as living a sedentary lifestyle. If you're reading this, you obviously don't want to be in that category. Being a pretty active guy, 10k is no sweat for me. Through my daily routine and exercise regimen, I easily surpass this amount. I set 15,000 for my personal goal, but often reach 20k. You don't have to do the same but you do have to learn to measure your steps, set a goal, and then gradually surpass that goal. Remaining stagnant is no longer an option for you. You want a healthier version of yourself and you will be able to achieve it! Measure it and get it done!

4. Weigh yourself everyday

In the spirit of measuring things, you must weigh yourself everyday. Can that number be a bit of a shock at first? Of course it can be! But weighing yourself daily gives you an understanding of your starting point and keeps you honest. I like to weigh myself first thing in the morning after I have gone to the bathroom. Weigh yourself without clothes, at the same time every day. You want to be consistent. There are a number of scales that you can use to keep yourself motivated while measuring your weight.

FitBit, the same company that makes the fitness trackers, makes a scale that connects wirelessly to your Internet. This scale also offers a method of measuring body fat. Measuring body fat is a complicated process and electronic scales can only be so accurate. Regardless it's another data point that can help you understand your current status. Additionally, this kind of scale uploads the information to your FitBit account and consolidates all the data with your step and activity information. Again it's another way to measure your activity and as we said earlier, what gets measured gets understood and gets done. I have found that weighing myself on a daily basis keeps me from straying too far from my target weight and allows me to modify my diet and activity to compensate depending where the scale is going. I also understand that weight fluctuates daily depending on water and a number of other factors. So I don't get too upset if I am off a pound or two from one day to the next. The most important thing is to watch out for the trends and catch any significant weight shifts.

5. Learn to love to move

Through my new fitness mantra of moving or losing, I feel compelled to stay in motion. That doesn't mean I'm constantly moving but it does mean that I am rarely on the coach for long periods of time. Being stuck in a car for an hour or even taking a flight drives me crazy! Having read so many studies that show how detrimental sitting is, I want to do the most that I can to stay moving. But it's beyond that. I find that many people who begin a fitness program do so with good intentions but do not engage in the correct mindset. You have to learn to love to move and be active. If you are coming from a mental place of hating to move, stand, walk, or workout, then you will increase your chances of failure. Instead, embrace your natural movement! The human body is an amazing vessel capable of inspiring things. But you don't have to be an athlete to unleash this natural ability. Enjoy moving for it makes you feel good, look good, and keeps your body working optimally. Everything else will follow from that. This tip is very much connected to tip #1. Physical fitness is as much as a result of proper mental focus as anything else.

6. Walk 30 minutes every day

By walking for 30 minutes every day, you will begin to solidify your habit of moving and be on your way to completing your 10k step daily goal. I prefer walking outside whenever possible because of the added benefit of fresh air, being outside, exposure to natural light, and the feeling of actual ground beneath your feet. When walking outside isn't possible, then a treadmill or indoor mall will do. You will need comfortable sneakers. I recommend getting running shoes that fit you properly. You may want to visit a sneaker store that can capture video of you walking. By doing this, the sneaker specialist can advise you on proper shoes. You want proper shoes that fit your feet to make walking comfortable and to avoid any possible injury. If you haven't been walking, try 10 minutes at first, and gradually increase. You eventually want to increase your time and then of course, your intensity. Your walking need not be of speed variety, but you should eventually be walking fast enough to elevate your heart rate a bit. If 30 minutes seems too much, you can break it into sessions during the day. And if you have a dog, you now have another reason to get out there!

I try walking for about an hour every day with my dog Buffy. We both get outside and our physical activity. I love nature and feel like I'm giving my dog that same gift. We both sleep soundly as an added side effect of this activity. Anything you can use as motivation is a plus!

7. Add more intense exercise sessions 3x per week

As you begin to get more comfortable with your 10,000 steps a day goal, you can then begin to add even more intense exercise sessions. As always, when starting exercise routine you must know your own limits. There are things like understanding the difference between sore muscles or more significant pain that could be indicating a serious problem. For example, when I begin jogging on the treadmill I get soreness in my shins. It took a while to understand that this was part of the process of my body adapting to new stimulus. But you have to learn to listen to your body. Don't fear muscle soreness for that is a signal that your body is working in the building and to getting to adapt to your new stimulus. However, you need to understand the difference between muscle soreness from exercise and a pain that can signal something's potentially damaging. That's why it's smart to begin any exercise routine slowly and gradually add more intensity. This way, you can prevent injury while preparing your body for more challenges in the future.

If you are completely new to exercise and have been inactive for a long period of time then you probably should get a physical. The medical community suggests that Americans get an annual physical to measure blood levels, cholesterol, blood pressure, and weight. This is something I never miss. I wonder how many ailments and diseases could be prevented or at least dealt with sooner if more people would go for annual checkups. I also wonder of the increased benefits if physicals were even more comprehensive and preventative.

Now back to the intense exercise sessions. What is intense exercise? Well it can be different things for different people. Everyone begins at a different level. Breaking a sweat usually indicates a sustained period of exercise or exertion. When I go for my hour-long daily walks I don't really break a sweat. My pulse is elevated for sustained period of time however I don't get that intense level of exercise that I require. Still, adding intensity to your daily routine is not as challenging as it might appear.

If you enjoy walking, then turn your walks into something more intense. You can add ankle weights, you can swing your arms, and/or you can increase your speed. You can also do intervals in which you pick up your walking pace for 10 to 20 seconds and then you bring them back to your normal rate for a few minutes and repeat the cycle. The point is if you get your heart rate elevated and that you break a sweat. These more intense exercise sessions will improve muscle tone, cardiovascular health, and your overall mood.

Measuring your pulse is a good way to determine whether or not you are exercising intensely enough. You can do this informally or you can use a device that can track it. Personally, I find having to wear a sensor around my chest to be annoying. But technologies improving all the time so one can imagine that the new fitness trackers will be able to measure pulse effectively and accurately. This is just another way in which you can get a more definitive point of measurement to try to understand whether not you were exercising intensely enough.

Another factor to consider as you begin a fitness program is that your body adjusts to exercise quickly. Meeting at accustomed to your moment. So if you are pursuing various goals you will have to adjust as you proceed. If you are just beginning an exercise program you will see that within the first couple weeks and even months you will lose weight rapidly. Couple that with the change in diet and you should really see dramatic results. But as you start to reduce the weight, your body will become accustomed and will need increased stimulus. Regardless of your fitness goals, adding intense exercise three times a week is a wonderful gift you can give yourself. And remember that these tips or are designed to give you ideas on how to be more active. Give the gift of greater health to yourself by beginning someplace.

As you get stronger, you can begin experimenting with different programs. Jogging will increase the amount of energy you expend. Running is an excellent calorie burner. And once you feel comfortable jogging, you can then graduate to running. If running is too strenuous for you then there are other options at your disposal. Swimming is a wonderful and joint friendly exercise. You may want to take up a dance class or even Zumba. The beauty of beginning a stand, step, and walk habit is that once this initial lifestyle change takes root, then more significant changes will be less difficult to adopt. Find what you enjoy and then do a three times a week. If you get bored, try something new. There are so many different options and the world is your oyster. The bottom line: add exercise 3x per week at an intensity that is greater that your usual walking.

8. Stand up more

Did you know that the average American watches anywhere between four and six hours of television a day? If you're sleeping for 6 to 8 hours a day, working for another eight hours, and watching TV for another two, that does not very much time at all to be active. It should come as no surprise that there are so many overweight and unfit Americans today. Now, I understand that life is stressful and that there are many obstacles to healthy living. But I have found that being active helps reduce the stresses that are in my life. It helps me to be a more positive person. So I highly recommend finding ways to be more active in your daily life.

Some occupations are better than others to promote physical activity. For example, when I worked at a financial services firm, I was at my desk for most of the day. I had to answer calls and I had to be at my computer terminal for most of it. So I would adapt. With my backup partner in place, I would get up to see a supervisor. I would take some time to talk to my colleagues. My job wasn't conducive to movement but I found ways around it. I would have lunch and then get up and walk around. [As an aside, I think that it is insane for worker to eat lunch trapped at their desks. Take the time to get away, enjoy your lunch, and walk around a little before tackling the rest of the day's work!] I would use my traveling on the subway as an opportunity for walking as I would often times walk all the way down to the end of the train in order to get more activity. The point is that there are ways to increase your daily movement even if you have a relatively sedentary job.

When I became a high school teacher, I found that being active was easier. Having my fitness tracker gave me insight. It was not uncommon by the time I return home that I would have accumulated 6-8 thousand steps for the day. I achieved this by adopting one of my favorite teacher practices for classroom management: walking around the classroom. My students must of thought I was a bit of a lunatic as I was marching up and down the isles but I enjoyed it. Walking around the room allowed me to interact more effectively with my students and put me in the "zone." And as a wonderful side effect I was able to remain active and boost my step count. There were times when I would take a stroll through the halls after eating my lunch to digest and enjoy the energy of the school community doing its thing.

Now that I have a home office, I have found new ways to remaining active. While I am writing I use a software dictation program to translate my voice into physical text. This allows me to stand up while I'm working. To boost my physical activity I actually march in place for most of this time as I'm writing. Now this may be eccentric for some people but let me explain.

Marching in place is a wonderful tool for increasing physical activity. It is not strenuous, it doesn't require any tools, and it does not require for you to actually get any piece of equipment, or get outside. And best of all, you can employ it while completing a variety of tasks during the day. The applications of marching in place are limitless. Of course, you won't find me doing this in public as some people may question your sanity. Being home and in private, your health is completely in your hands and what you do to enhance it is really up to you. One of the things that allows me to boost my daily steps is my everyday movement. By marching in place, I can boost the steps and I achieve my goals - often surpassing them by using this technique. I have found great success by using this marching in place in conjunction with one of my favorite activities. Which leads me to...

9. March in place while you watch TV – crazy perhaps, but effective

This is one habit that I keep to myself – until now... Some family members think that I'm crazy for doing this. Many people believe that watching television is pure relaxation and escapism. Sometimes, zoning out on the couch in front of the television is a great stress relief. But this comes at a cost. By sitting down for hours at a time, you deactivate your body. Your nervous system decreases in activity as your body realizes that you are not going to demand much of it during this time.

Now, I do love my television. I'm a big fan of pop culture and always have been. Currently there are about 7 to 10 programs on my TiVo recorder. I make no apologies for it. I enjoy it. But I also want an active lifestyle and realize that every hour I am on the couch is an hour that I am not working on keeping myself healthy.

There is an added benefit to marching in place while watching television. I zone out too when I watch TV. If it's something really good, then I usually stop paying attention to everything else. This is a prime example of retraining your mind! There are times where I am watching television and go marching in place and when I finally checked my fitness tracker I found that this added 4000-5000 steps to my daily total! This amount of steps is halfway to the goal of 10,000 a day. There are other ways to adopt this practice. For example, in the course of an hour program, let's say you stand up and march and place during the commercial break. This way you can ease yourself into the concept of marching in place while watching television. Yes, watching television has always been connected to relaxation. And sometimes you will need to just to sit on the couch and relax. I understand this and grant myself this little slice of sedentary relaxation.

But I hope that you'll come to understand that the more you are active during your day, and the more you stand, step, and walk, you can really make dramatic improvements to your health.

10. Add resistance training

To the novice exerciser, resistance training may seem a bit challenging. But it really isn't. The one caveat to resistance training is that you're not actually doing too much stepping. That's one of the reasons I sometimes don't enjoy resistance training as much as a good walk or run –it doesn't really add to my step count!

Still, the scientific research shows that resistance training has amazing benefits.[11] Adding resistance training to your routine builds lean muscle, which increases your metabolism. Adding weights to your exercise program also strengthens muscles and joints making injury less likely any other activities. I strongly believe that in addition to a good and constant stand, step, and walk routine, resistance training is vital to a healthy lifestyle.

I recommend beginning a resistance-training program with bodyweight exercises. Bodyweight squats and push-ups are two excellent exercises. There are ways to modify these exercises if they are too challenging at first. For example, use a chair while doing your bodyweight squats. You can simply sit in a chair and stand up and repeat that until you feel strong enough to squat without the chair. As for the push-up (the king of bodyweight exercises for the upper body), you can modify it by doing push-ups on your knees so you're not lifting your entire body weight. If you're interested in beginning bodyweight exercises there are many resources on the web that can teach you with videos on how to safely and properly use your body as the ultimate training tool.

Other obvious way to begin resistance training is to use actual weights. You can join a gym or start a home gym. I invested in an adjustable weight dumbbell set which allows me to use to do a variety of exercises at different levels of weight. If you feel apprehensive because this is new to you, I recommend seeking out a personal trainer who can instruct you. If you start slowly and with light weights, the risk of injury is relatively low. However you must always use proper form and if you're not sure of the proper form then consult a professional or at least read up on it. I will tell you that from my experience the only time I've injured myself is when I did not follow the rules and increased the amount of weight beyond what was the normal progression. Other than that, the only discomfort I only felt from resistance training is the soreness that follows. But as we discussed earlier, soreness is natural in the process and good for you and your healthier lifestyle.

Summary

Adopting a stand, step, and walk routine is just the beginning on your life long journey of healthy living. Once you cultivate a habit of being more active, you will begin to see changes in your body and feel clarity in your mind and attitudes. And as you become more active, you will want to do things that increase your daily activity. By using a fitness tracker, you can actually measure and understand your daily activity. This is one of the most important steps to begin your healthy living transformation. But getting more active will only get you so far in your journey. Next I'll share what I've learned about nutrition and healthy eating.

5. Nutrition and food intake – your partners to a healthier you

Now that you've explored ways to add more activity in your life, you can now begin to understand the other partners in healthy living – nutrition and healthy eating.

There is a ton of information on this area and sometimes it may even seem contradictory. I will share what I have learned from my own experiences and it is simple: eat less.

Earlier, I wrote of how my Dad recommended that I just eat half of what I would normally eat to lose weight. He was so right. While I chose to use Weight Watchers® and its mobile app, the concept was the same. I had to recalibrate what was normal in the amount of food that I was eating. That huge peanut butter and jelly bagel became a half. That three serving of breakfast cereal became one. Those three slices of pizza became a single slice of heaven. The key point is that I don't deprive myself of the foods I love – I just am conscious of how much I eat of them.

You can get very technical in this area by calculating your resting metabolic rate and factoring in your age and lifestyle. That's fine and you may want to do that. But I find that simplicity is closest to the truth – portion control. This is something that I didn't want to consider for the longest time. I used food as a substitute for entertainment and for even emotional eating. Until we realize that food is merely the way we sustain ourselves and treat it as such, there is a danger that we will continue to overindulge in too large portions. Another minefield is eating out. Huge portions of delicious food that you didn't have to prepare is a temptation many cannot resist. You may think that your selection of chicken and brown rice may be a healthy one, until to start to calculate the calories of your portion.

That is why I found Weight Watchers®[12] so effective. For the first couple of weeks (annoying) I had to measure everything I ate. Those two tablespoons of peanut butter were counted as five points. My daily total when I began was 41 (now I'm at a daily total of 29) and five precious points went to that sometimes two times a day indulgence. So measuring something makes you consider the cost/benefit of consuming it. I know to use a teaspoon rather than tablespoon to measure out my peanut butter. And while I reduced that amount of eat of it, I can never imagine my life without the creamy and rich flavor of peanut butter.

At what level you begin your calorie restriction depends on number of factors. As you already know, I am not a nutritionist nor medical doctor. But I have read extensively and can use my own experience as a baseline. There are a number of ways to formulate exactly what your daily caloric needs and how much you need to reduce your calories are to begin losing weight. There are a number of weight-loss tools that can help you calculate this. You can go as simple as eating ¼ less of what you eat normally. This is an easy way to visualizing on the food you eat in your plate and simply cut it by one fourth. Or you want to get more exact and actually calculate your body's metabolic needs and then use that number as a baseline. I have used a very good and free app called MyFitnessPal[13]. This provides you with great information such as the amount of calories and macronutrients in practically every food you can consume. By using this tool or others you may get a better understanding of your caloric needs.

The principle to use in order to understand your daily food consumption is to keep a food journal. By actually taking the time to write down the food that you're eating, you begin to realize exactly when putting into your body. This is another reason why the Weight Watchers app or MyFitnessPal can be very useful to your healthy lifestyle. These apps use the principle of a food diary by encouraging you to look up food and record what and how much you eat of it. Keeping a food diary is a powerful habit that makes you aware. Simplicity can provide you with the best results. By being honest about what you're eating, writing it down, and reflecting, you can begin to me tremendous advances in your health and overall fitness.

I strongly recommend that you begin to be more aware of what and how much you eat. Once you start to do this, you will see patterns emerge and hopefully begin to make better choices.

I like to address a final note on eating. A proper diet is one that involves natural foods that are minimally processed. Eating these kinds of foods and in the proper portions will allow you to lose weight and maintain a healthy level of weight effortlessly. Still, I am a big believer in enjoying life and delicious food is a big part of that. And for many of us, having all good food all the time can be boring. We sometimes want a slice of cake, a scoop of ice cream, a piece of dark chocolate (healthy in small portions too), or a piece of candy. Sometimes we need that cheeseburger and fries (one of my favorite meals). I have found that if you can eat well roughly 80% of the time you can enjoy these foods. It is all about balance. You can't eat a cheeseburger and fries every day – that's just common sense. But you don't have to eat celery sticks and tiny teaspoons of almond butter all the time either. I like to adhere to a healthy diet for six days of the week and I will choose one day I'll splurge a little bit. Now as you will reduce your food intake and start to lose weight, you will find that you can't eat as much as he used to. This alone acts as a natural limitation of how much you can eat. I have found that my stomach just can't hold a large capacity anymore. Even on my cheat days, my body regulates how many additional calories I could possibly consume. Again, I don't deprive myself of anything that I want. The only rule is to eat healthy and portion control for most of the time and then you can enjoy your occasional indulgence.

And as always, eat more vegetables than fruits. Reduce your consumption of white flour and related products. Consume small amount of healthy fats. Lean protein is your friend. A portion-controlled diet comprised of those food items will help you zoom towards to your health and fitness goals.

6. All hands on deck
How simple public policy and healthcare changes could encourage Americans to live healthier

Healthcare Industry

I am an advocate for free markets and the healthcare market is not exempt from my views. With healthcare costs rising every year in United States, isn't about time that we took a look at the healthcare market and how we can improve it? I think that most people can agree that high quality and affordable healthcare for as many people as possible is a worthwhile goal for any civilized society. But looking at today's system, can we conclude that it works as cost-effective and as fairly as it could? I surely do not. But I thought about how the healthcare industry and insurance industry works and I've come up with some easy solutions that I think could help tremendously.

1. Open and fair pricing

I always saw insurance as a method of protecting oneself against catastrophic events. Get into a car accident and obviously insurance can be very important. With a good insurance policy, damage to your home can be repaired. But these events should be few and far between. I never understood why a routine physical must be covered by insurance. When the blood work must be covered by insurance. How about letting people be responsible for their normal physical monitoring? The medical community suggests that everyone should get a yearly physical. That's reasonable to me and all seems reasonable that people should pay for that physical rather than pushing a lot of the cost onto the insurance companies. Just as retailers display their pricing and have sales and the like, doctors and medical providers across the nation should be open and clear on what they charge for their services. The more important point is that doctors and patients if allowed could negotiate better pricing for health care.

2. An ounce of prevention...

It boggles the mind why healthcare providers and insurance companies do not focus more on preventative care. I will provide a personal example. A couple years ago my father went to the bathroom to urinate. That usual routine act provided a great shock to him. Blood was in his urine. After a number of tests and valuation it was determined that my father had stage III kidney cancer. Thankfully, he had access to terrific doctors who were able to remove the kidney and to this day my father is cancer free.

Still, a physical that would've included an MRI or CAT scan could have potentially caught the cancer years ago. But as you probably are aware, an MRI or CAT scan are not considered part of routine physical care for most people. I understand these are expensive tests but the cost of these tests could have easily been less then the treatment that was required for my father once the kidney cancer was discovered. Now my father's over fifty, and I can see the wisdom of preventative tests for adults his age and over. More aggressive focus on preventative care by the medical community could save lives, and reduce healthcare costs for all.

3. Encourage healthier lifestyles
      I am a big believer the medical community and health insurance industry could do a much better job and encouraging healthy lifestyles. While is difficult to convince people to change their habits, a concerted and coordinated effort by the medical community and insurance companies could sustain gradual and important change in many people's lives. As discussed, fitness trackers are terrific tools for personal use. Where are the programs to provide people with fitness trackers and incentivize their use? One company does a tremendous job doing this is Walgreens. By connecting your Walgreens account with a fitness tracker (like a FitBit), you can be awarded balance points on your account. These points can then be redeemed for dollars amounts toward your bill at Walgreens. When I found out about this I jumped on it. I thought it was an excellent way to reward people for a healthier lifestyle or healthy lifestyle choices. Of course it works with human nature and the desire to be rewarded for one's actions. An excellent business decision becomes a wonderful gift to promoting healthier lifestyles. Even some insurance companies are beginning to develop programs to incentivize healthier habits. For example, Oscar Health Insurance will provide its members with Amazon.com gift cards for the number of steps they take.[14]

Government policy

      I'm a big believer that government tends to get into the way of many areas of our daily lives. As such, the majority of my recommendations are for government to let the market work fairly and more efficiently.

1. Allow for insurance companies to sell across state lines
      Through arcane law, insurance companies cannot sell across state lines. If insurance companies could sell policies across state lines to more people, then rates of insurance could drop. This is a no brainer issue for the government to adjust.

2. Decouple health insurance from employment
      I strongly disagree with having employers provide health insurance. Yes, many employers do shoulder a lot of the cost but that is not without another cost: to the employee. Businesses and employers select health insurance plans and often times these plans can be not in the best interest of all employees. At the same time, having employers provide health insurance lowers wages and removes responsibility from where it should be – the individual. And while this is a significant change to the current way that health insurance is provided for majority of people, I think it will encourage greater competition enhanced choice for many individuals.

3. Reduce fraud and frivolous lawsuits

Federal and local agencies should investigate and prosecute fraud across healthcare. This includes insurance fraud as well as Medicare and Medicaid fraud as well. State and federal judiciaries should take steps to limit frivolous lawsuits that add to the cost of practicing and providing medical care. Let acts of carelessness and negligence be punished but also punish those who are seeking to defraud the system in the quest of a quick buck.

By implementing these and other simple reforms, the quality of health and healthcare in America would improve. Society would be in greater shape if we would restore individual decisions and responsibility to, gasp, the individual! People taking charge of their own health and the health of their families would lead to wonderful improvements across the nation. And once the healthcare industry and government are more properly aligned with that main principle, then people will have an easier task of becoming healthier. Let us remove the obstacles to healthy living.

7. Conclusion
Stand, Step, and walk yourself to a healthier you

Without good health, we can have all the success, money, family, and friends in the world but then we couldn't really enjoy those things. Therefore, we all need to take responsibility for our health by making better choices and cultivating positive habits.

I wrote *Stand, Step, and Walk Yourself to a Healthier You* because of my love for health and fitness and my desire to inform and motivate people to love it too. Healthier living should not be a burden. It is a life long commitment to keep you running in peak condition. By making simple changes in our minds and choosing habits that will support our goals, everyone can achieve a healthier lifestyle.

So decide to get healthier. Create the proper mindset and increase your willpower. Make small changes. Stand more. Step more. Walk more. Measure your activity so you can motivate yourself to continue on this path. Reduce your food intake and choose healthier food options but never deprive yourself (as long as you do it occasionally). Exercise more. Get up at the office. Walk to a coworker instead of sending that email. Park your car further away from the supermarket or mall – walk that extra distance. Take the time to enjoy life. Healthy living isn't really a sacrifice. It's a way to live so that you can keep yourself happy, healthy, and energetic for yourself and all those people you love in your life. Yes, looking good naked is a happy side effect of a healthier lifestyle too. But you want to have a high quality life, then health is key. Prevent many common ailments and age related issues. You get one body. You get one life. Do what is in your control to influence your life and your health. Be responsible.

Stand, step, and walk yourself to a healthier you.

Sources & Notes

[1] *The Facts About Emotional Eating*. CNN. http://www.cnn.com/2012/10/03/living/real-simple-emotional-eating/index.html

[2] *Adult Obesity facts*. CDC. http://www.cdc.gov/obesity/data/adult.html

[3] *Adult Obesity facts*. CDC. http://www.cdc.gov/obesity/data/adult.html

[4] *Heart Disease facts*. CDC. http://www.cdc.gov/heartdisease/facts.htm

[5] *Risks of physical inactivity*. John Hopkins Medicine. http://www.hopkinsmedicine.org/healthlibrary/conditions/cardiovascular_diseases/risks_of_physical_inactivity_85,P00218/

[6] Servan-Schreiber, David, MD. *Anticancer*. Viking: 2009.

[7] Juststand.org

[8] Rath, Tom. *Eat Move Sleep*. Missionday: 2013.

[9] Adams, Susan. *New Study: Treadmill desks boost productivity*. Forbes. March 2014.

[10] Study: 10,000 Steps A Day is Good for You. Fox News. 2012. http://www.foxnews.com/story/2010/02/22/study-10000-steps-day-is-good-for/

[11] WebMD. http://www.webmd.com/fitness-exercise/features/get-more-burn-from-your-workout

[12] I do not endorse Weight Watchers® or the company's products. I merely have used its program and found its principles to be effective for weight loss and maintenance.

[13] I do not endorse, work, or profit from MyFitnessPal.

[14] Humer, Caroline. *New York health insurer Oscar to pay members who walk more*. 2014. http://www.reuters.com/article/2014/12/08/us-usa-healthcare-oscar-idUSKBN0JM25F20141208